RECIPES 4
R A W   F O O D

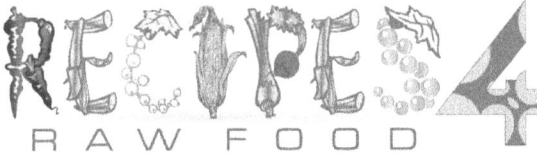

20 Awesome Raw Appetizers You Can't Live Without

By Kathy Tennefoss

Raw Food Recipes & Tips for Living a Healthy Life!

MEMBER OF THE RAW FOODS ASSOCIATION

RECIPES 4
R A W   F O O D

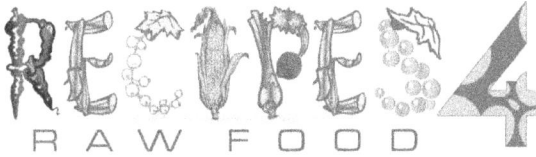

20 Awesome Raw Appetizers Food You Can't Live
Without

Sunny Cabana Publishing, L.L.C.

Fort Lauderdale, FL

www.sunnycabanapublishing.com

By Kathy Tennefoss

Published by Kathleen Tennefoss
Printed in the United States of America
Author: Kathy Tennefoss
Editor: Shawn M Tennefoss
13-digit ISBN: 9781936874101
10-digit ISBN: 1936874105
First Printing

This book is dedicated to my dad James Kelley for pushing me in the right direction regarding healthy eating, living a healthy active life, and to my loving husband Shawn Tennefoss for suffering through my computer difficulties and taking the time to show me how to orchestrate this book along with sharing his life and journey with me.

Cover design: Kathy & Shawn Tennefoss

First edition, 2011

Acknowledgements:

Thanks to everyone who encouraged and inspired me and gave me excellent input and feedback in the raw food industry, including one of my many sisters Heather McNerney, my husband Shawn M. Tennefoss, my dad James Kelley, and Melissa Hernandez and her wonderful family! Without everyone's input I would not have finished this book or started other raw food recipe books. I am extremely grateful to everyone.

If you have any suggestions, comments, or corrections please send me an email to recipes4rawfood@yahoo.com.

Disclaimer:
The responsibility for any adverse detoxification effects resulting from using these recipes described lies not with the author or distributors of this book. This book is not intended for medical advice just as suggestion. Please enjoy these recipes with your friends and family.

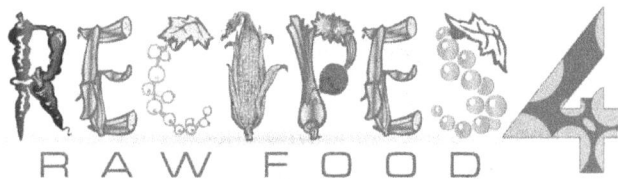

RECIPES 4
R A W   F O O D

Table of Contents

Intro

Today you hear "I'm too busy and I don't have time to eat healthy or it costs too much". Well I'm here to say that it only takes a few minutes to have a healthy meal. For the time it takes to go to the drive through and wait in line to have some high fat low nutrition meal you can make a quick raw meal. If cost is your concern buy your organic produce in bulk or choose an organic buying club that delivers produce weekly to your home. You don't have to eat this way everyday but you will feel a huge difference in your body just after a few days of eating this way. Your skin will start to feel better, your clothes will be fitting loser, and you might even have more energy! Isn't that worth it!

This book on raw appetizers is a small window into the raw food arena. It is nice to prepare raw appetizers for small gatherings to get people used to the taste, experience, and idea of raw food. With bite size pieces everyone gets to try it! People will be amazed at the taste and will want to eat dinner at your house e all the time. This could become a problem but at least everyone will be eating a healthy diet!

Please try to use as much organic produce as possible when making your raw recipes or any other meal you plan to prepare. Starting with the freshest ingredients is always the best option plus they taste better and you're helping the environment by purchasing local organic ingredients.

A Ripe Juicy Tomato - an Incredibly Tasty and Healthy Treat

There is nothing more satisfying than enjoying a fresh, ripe, juicy tomato at the peak of the growing season. Sure, you can purchase tomatoes year round in the grocery store, and some of them are tasty, but there is much to be said for growing your own tomatoes and enjoying the fruits of your labor right off the vine.

Not only do homegrown fruits and vegetables taste great, but by growing your own raw food, you can enjoy organic fruits and vegetables without the worry of hazardous chemicals and pesticides.

Not only do fresh raw tomatoes taste good, they are good for you, too. Raw food such as fruits and vegetables boast of many health and beauty benefits. Here are a few things to feel good about when you enjoy eating delicious juicy raw tomatoes.

The Tomato / Cancer Connection

My friend has an amazing garden and grows some incredible tomatoes in the summer months. She often gives me tips and pointers for my own garden. She doesn't allow people to smoke in her garden because she says it will harm the tomato plants. There are mixed thoughts on this subject, but she stands her ground adamantly.

Well, guess what? Smoking might not be good for tomatoes, but tomatoes are good for smoking. They contain two acids that fight against the carcinogens created by cigarette smoke.

The tomato doesn't stop there in its war against cancer. The lycopene pigment found in tomatoes contributes to fewer chances of prostate cancer, colorectal cancer, and stomach cancer. Lycopene is somewhat of a miracle ingredient that scientists believe stops cancer cells from growing.

Tomatoes Even Make You Pretty

Tomatoes are high in vitamin A, which is a great benefit for many reasons. First, vitamin A improves vision and most notably helps with night blindness, but the mighty A does more than help your eyesight. The vitamin A in tomatoes also supports shiny hair, good bones, vibrant skin, and healthy teeth.

Vitamin A combines with the vitamin C in tomatoes to provide a strong anti-oxidant defense against free radicals in the blood. Some of the beta-carotene produced by these two vitamins is lost in cooking because it destroys the vitamin C, which is why a raw tomato snack is a good choice.

Raw Tomatoes are Healthy for Your Heart

Tomatoes contain niacin, potassium, and vitamin B6. Eating tomatoes can reduce cholesterol levels, help with high blood pressure, and lower your risk for heart disease.

While the traditional saying is that an apple a day keeps the doctor away, tomatoes should have their place in your healthy diet, too. By snacking on these delicious fruits often, you'll be doing something beneficial to your health, all while enjoying something so incredibly delicious as a fresh, ripe, juicy tomato.

SPICY SUN DRIED TOMATO & PABLANO DIP

1 dried pablano pepper soaked in a small amount of water
1 cup soaked raw cashews
¼ cup olive oil
1 cup soaked sundried tomatoes (keep the liquid from the soaked tomatoes)
Celtic salt and black pepper

Take the pablono pepper that has been soaked and drained. Take the pablano pepper, the drained cashews, olive oil, the sun dried tomatoes, and salt and pepper and put all of the ingredients in a vita mixer and blend until smooth. You will need to add some of the water back into the mixer until it blends smoothly. It just depends on how smooth you like the dip. Then use romaine leaves, carrots, cucumbers to dip.

TOMATO & AVACADO TOWER

3 Small orange tomatoes
3 Small Red Tomatoes

2 Avocados
Olive Oil
Balsamic Vinegar

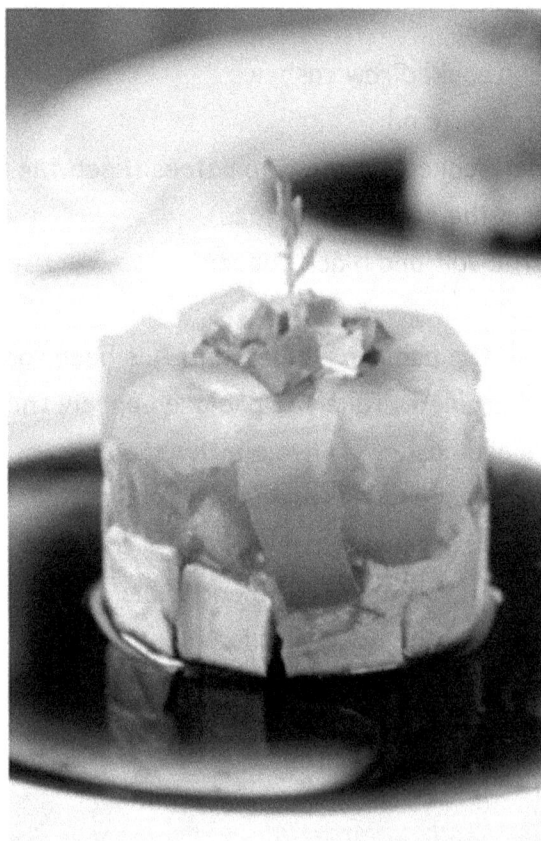

First take both types of tomatoes and chop into small pieces. Next take the avocados and scoop out the insides and chop into small pieces. Next take the avocado and place in a round area on your presentation plate. Then take the other tomatoes and layer them on the avocado in the shape of a tower. Now drizzle with olive oil and balsamic vinegar. Use the salt and pepper to your taste.

TROPICAL PLANTAIN SLAW

1 head of Napa cabbage shredded thinly
1 red pepper sliced thin
Sauce
1 really ripe plantain
1 orange peeled
$\frac{1}{2}$ cup almond butter
$\frac{1}{4}$ cup of olive oil
$\frac{1}{4}$ teaspoon of red pepper flakes
Celtic sea salt and black pepper to taste

Take the shredded cabbage and thinly sliced red peppers and put in a large bowl. Next take the ingredients for the sauce and blend

in a vita mixer until smooth with a medium
consistency and then pour the sauce on the
cabbage and red peppers and mix well. You
can use this slaw for a filling in collard
greens, large romaine leaves, or just by
itself.

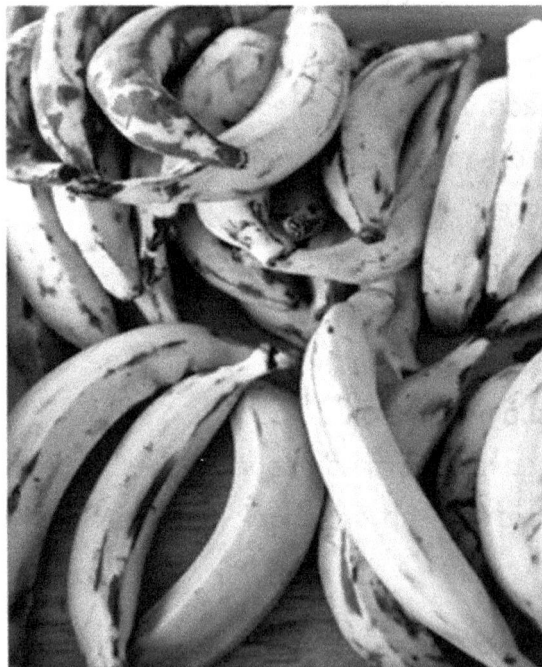

CILANTRO PESTO DIP

1 cup cilantro
½ cup olive oil
2 tablespoon hemp oil
1 cup of pumpkin seeds soaked
Celtic sea salt and black pepper

Mix all ingredients in a vita mixer until smooth. You may want to save some of the water from the pumpkin seeds that were soaking to use to smooth out the dip. The consistency should be a medium consistency. You can use this pesto to dip your veggies in or as a base for your wraps. Either way this is a yummy dip!

MARINATED MUSHROOMS
3 cups of sliced mushrooms of every variety that you like (portabella and crimini work well)
1/8 cup of olive oil
1 tablespoon of vinegar of your choice
1 teaspoon of agave nectar

1 teaspoon of Braggs
Celtic sea salt and black pepper
1 clove of garlic diced small
1 teaspoon of cumin

Take all of the liquid ingredients and marinate the mushrooms in the sauce overnight. Then you can use these mushrooms for dipping in sauces, raw pizzas, or just by themselves!

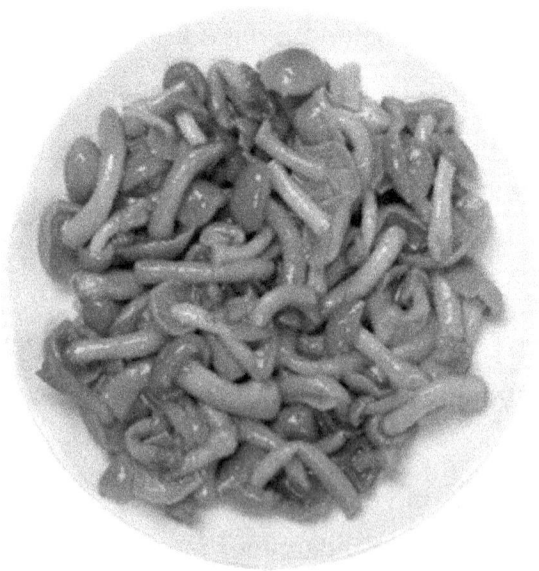

TOMATO, ONION, & PARM CAPRESE

1-2 large tomatoes
1 sweet onion
Olive oil and balsamic for the top
$\frac{1}{4}$ cup chopped basil

Parm
$\frac{1}{2}$ cup cashews
$\frac{1}{2}$ cup pine nuts
1 clove of garlic
$\frac{1}{2}$ teaspoon of Braggs
3 tablespoons of nutritional yeast
2 tablespoons of lemon juice
Celtic sea salt
Take and slice the tomatoes and onions in
rounds. Next take the pine nuts, cashews,
nutritional yeast, garlic, lemon juice, salt,
and Braggs and mix in a vita mixer until the
mixture is fine. Take the sliced tomatoes
and sliced onions and tower them on top of
each other and sprinkle them with the
parmesan and sprinkle with olive oil,
balsamic, and basil.

MANGO SALSA

1 large mango peeled and sliced into small
pieces
2 limes
1 cup of cilantro
1 hass avocado diced
1 small jalapeño
1 teaspoon of olive oil
$\frac{1}{2}$ red peppers
Celtic salt and black pepper

Take the mango and mix in the juice of the
limes, chopped cilantro, diced avocado,
jalapeño diced small, and diced red pepper
and mix together with 1 teaspoon of olive oil
and salt and pepper. Use this for a dip with
raw crackers or as a sauce in wraps.

VEGETABLE TORTE

2 green zucchini
2 yellow zucchini

1 cup marinated mushrooms (from this section)
Raw ricotta
1 cup macadamia nuts soaked (save the soaked water)
3 tablespoons of nutritional yeast
$\frac{1}{4}$ cup lemon juice
Celtic sea salt and black pepper to taste

Blend the macadamia nuts with the lemon juice and enough water to make the mixture smooth, and then add the nutritional yeast, salt and pepper.

Take the zucchini's and slice very thin and alternate between marinated mushrooms and ricotta and the zucchini slices until all of the ingredients are gone. Then let set in the refrigerator for 1 hour and then serve with raw crackers or by it!
Thai noodles

2 young coconuts
$\frac{1}{2}$ cup of almond butter

1 lime
1 small banana
1 teaspoon yellow curry (if you want green or
red is fine also; it depends on your taste)
$\frac{1}{2}$ cup of cilantro
$\frac{1}{4}$ cup Thai basil
1-2 Thai peppers

Take the young coconuts and scoop the
young coconut out and be sure to be careful
to not break it up too much. Then take the
coconut and slice it thinly so that it looks
like noodles. In another bowl take the $\frac{1}{2}$ cup
of the coconut water, small banana, almond
butter, juice of the lime, curry, and salt and
pepper and mix until smooth. Take this
sauce and pour it over the coconut noodles
and then garnish with basil, cilantro, and
sliced Thai peppers (it depends on how hot
you like it so use accordingly) yum.

MUSHROOM PATE

1 cup of almonds that have been soaked
1 cup of raw sunflower seeds soaked
2 tablespoons of lemon juice
1 red pepper rough chopped
1 carrot chopped
1 cup cilantro
1 clove of garlic
$\frac{1}{4}$ onion chopped
$\frac{1}{4}$ cup nutritional yeast
1 cup of marinated mushrooms
1 tablespoon of Braggs

Take all of the ingredients and mix in a food processor until well mixed and put the ingredients in a glass dish and refrigerate for an hour or so until firm and then serve with raw crackers or veggies.

SPICY & CHEESY JICAMA FRIES WITH CREAMY TOMATO SAUCE

2 large jicama peeled and sliced in the shape of french fries.

¼ teaspoon of cayenne
1 teaspoon of paprika
Salt and pepper
1 tablespoon of lime juice
1 teaspoon of olive oil
2 tablespoons of nutritional yeast

Sauce
½ cup of raw cashews soaked
3 small roma tomatoes
1/8 cup of olive oil
1 tablespoon of maple syrup
Salt and pepper to taste

Take the sliced jicama and toss with spices and olive oil. Next take the sauce ingredients and mix in a vita mixer until thick like the consistency of ketchup. Now dip the jicama in the sauce and enjoy!

STUFFED MINI SWEET PEPPERS

8-10 mini red and yellow sweet peppers
1 cup of walnuts soaked

½ cup cilantro
Salt and pepper
2 tablespoons of nutritional yeast
1 carrot chopped
1 teaspoon of cumin
½ teaspoon of cayenne
1 tablespoon of lemon juice

Take everything but the red peppers and mix in the vita mixer and blend until mixed well. Take the sweet peppers and cut the tops off and fill them with the mixture and serve.

GUACAMOLE

3 Hass Avocados
¼ Cup Lime Juice
½ Cup diced tomatoes
1 Jalapeño
1 Clove of Garlic
1 Bunch of Cilantro
Salt and Pepper
1 teaspoon of cumin

$\frac{1}{2}$ teaspoon of cayenne

Scoop the avocado out of the shells. Next cut the jalapeño in half and take the seeds out. In a vita mixer take the rest of the ingredients except for the tomatoes and blend until smooth. Now add the chopped tomatoes and your ready for your raw burritos.

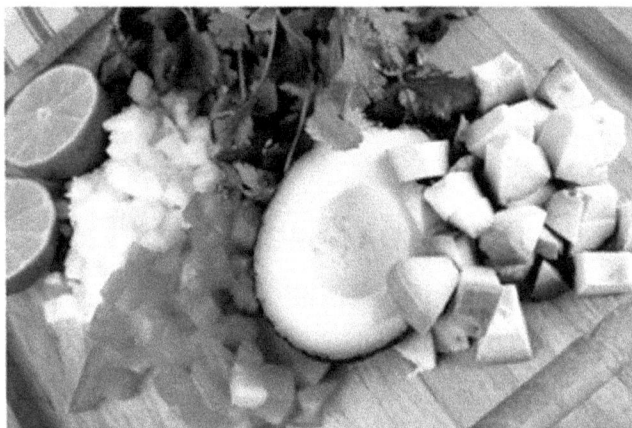

EASY SALSA

5 Tomatoes
$\frac{1}{2}$ Cup lime juice
1 Jalapeño

1 bunch of cilantro
½ small onion
1 clove of garlic
Salt and pepper
1 teaspoon of cumin
½ teaspoon of cayenne
1 cup chopped avocado

First take the jalapeño and cut in half and take the seeds out. Then take the rest of the ingredients except for the avocado and blend until choppy with a vita mixer. Now take the chopped avocados and mix them with the ingredients and serve with your favorite raw crackers!

GRAPEFRUIT, AVACADO, & BEET TOWER

2 Grapefruits
2 Avocados
2 beets
Small zucchini flowers

Micro greens
Salt and Pepper
Balsamic vinegar
Olive oil

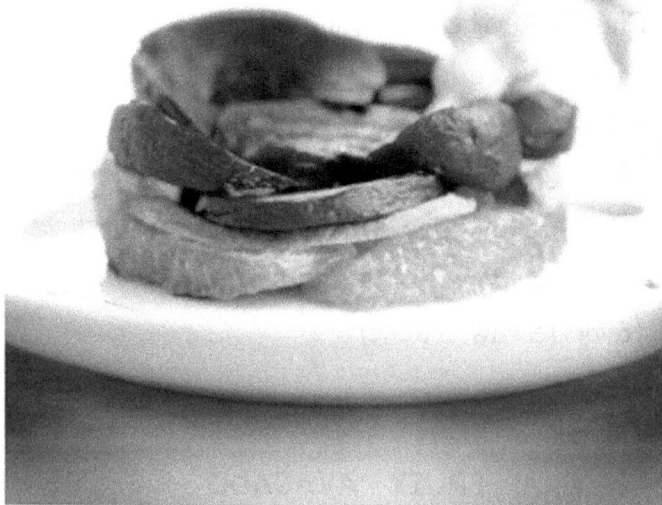

First take the grapefruit and peel them and
then slice them in a round circle. Next take
the avocados and scoop them out and chop
them in small pieces. For the final phase of

the tower take the two beets and peel them
and slice them really thin and marinate them
in with a little orange juice and Braggs for a
couple of hours.

Take one round grapefruit slice and add
some of the avocado to the top and then a
thin slice of the beet. Top with micro
greens and zucchini flowers and drizzle with
olive oil and balsamic vinegar. Keep doing this
until all the ingredients are used up for the
towers and serve.

JICAMA SALSA

1 Large Jicama
1 Red Pepper
1 Yellow Pepper
1 Orange
$\frac{1}{2}$ Cup Chopped Cilantro
Salt and Pepper

Take the jicama and peel it and chop into
small pieces. Next take the peppers and
take the seeds out and chop them also into

small pieces. Mix the jicama and peppers in a bowl and squeeze the juice of the orange onto the mixture. Now top with the cilantro and serve with dehydrated chips.

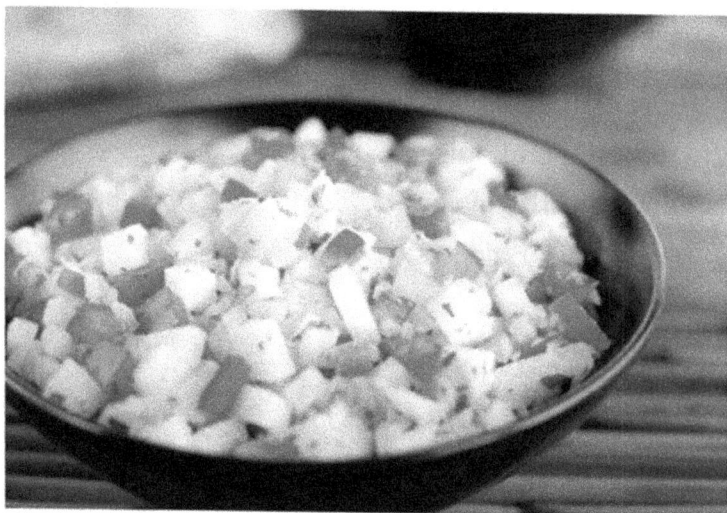

SPROUT & NORI WRAPS

Couple of large handfuls of sunflower sprouts
3 Nori Sheets
Nama Shoyu (raw soy sauce) for dipping

These are so simple and easy! First take the sunflower sprouts (or any sprouts that you prefer) and lay them in the nori sheets and wrap them up tight. Next slice them and place on a plate with the nama shoyu as a dipping sauce. You can use whatever sauce you like. Sometimes I will use an almond butter sauce made with a little almond butter and lime juice.

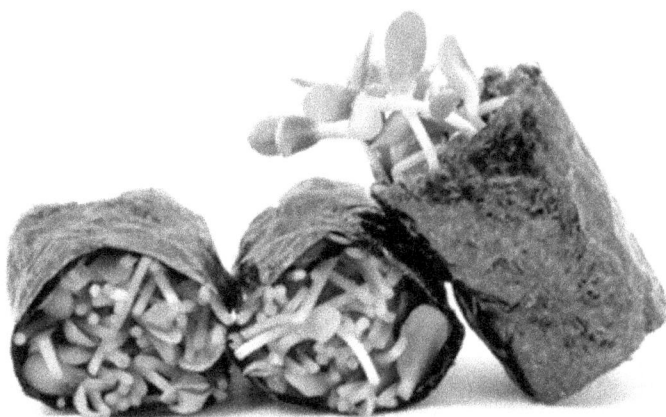

CHUNKY COWBOY CORN DIP

3 Ears of Corn
2 Tablespoons of Hemp Seeds
1 Large Red Pepper
½ Cup of Cilantro
Salt and Pepper to Taste
2 Tablespoons of lime juice
½ Teaspoon of cumin

First take the ears of corn and slice the corn off of the cob. Next take the red pepper and cut into small pieces. Mix the corn, red pepper, lime juice, s & p, cumin, and sprinkle with hemp seeds. You can eat this as a side salad or dip with raw crackers.

TANGY DILL DIP

1 Bunch of fresh dill
1 Cup of Cashews (soaked)
¼ cup of olive oil
1 Clove of garlic
2 Tablespoons of lime juice

$\frac{1}{2}$ teaspoon of sage

$\frac{1}{2}$ teaspoon of thyme

Salt & pepper

Take the soaked cashews and drain (save the liquid in case you may need it for a thinner sauce) and put in a vita mixer along with the rest of the ingredients and blend until smooth. Use on wraps or as a dip with raw chips.

COCONUT CURRY CARROT DIP

4 Medium carrots

1 Cup Macadamia nuts (soaked)

1 teaspoon curry powder

2 Tablespoons of coconut water

Basil for garnish

Salt and Pepper

Take the carrots and clean and peel them and put them in a vita mixer along with the

rest of the ingredients until smooth.
Garnish with the basil and serve.

VEGGY ANITPASTI

1 Cup of Marinated Portobello's
1 Small Eggplant
1 Red Pepper
$\frac{1}{2}$ Bunch of Asparagus
$\frac{1}{2}$ cup of balsamic vinegar
$\frac{1}{2}$-3/4 Cup of olive oil
2 small zucchini
Salt and Pepper

First take the eggplant and zucchini and
slice with a mandolin (or very fine). Then
slice the red pepper thinly and trim the
asparagus. Now take the above ingredients
and soak for 1 hour in the balsamic vinegar
and olive oil. Drain and place nicely on a
platter with raw chips and serve.

ABOUT THE AUTHOR:

B.S. Science in Physical Anthropology minor in business, and Culinary Arts Degree.

Advocate for organic, vegetarian, vegan, raw food diets, writing, yoga, swimming, biking, and running 5 K's! I have been a vegetarian/vegan/raw foodist for over 20 years. I have also worked in real estate for over ten years and have several websites to help people who are interested in raw food http://www.Recipes4RawFood.com and http://www.RawFoodForToday.com .

I have also started the Raw Foods Association with my husband so that others can become members of a larger healthy group and its website is www.RawFoodsAssociation.com!

For more information on how to order books, original articles, become a member of the Raw Foods Association, and updates on future projects go to www.rawfoodfortoday.com, www.recipes4rawfood.com, or www.sunnycabanapublishing.com.

RECIPES 4
R A W F O O D

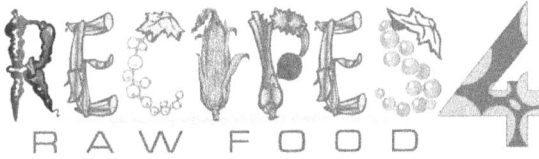

1314 E Las Olas Blvd

Fort Lauderdale, FL 33301

Recipes4RawFood@yahoo.com

I hope you enjoy my raw appetizer recipes!

Check out more of my recipes at
www.recipes4rawfood.com and
www.rawfoodfortoday.com

If you have any suggestions, comments, or corrections please feel free to email me at recipes4rawfood@yahoo.com.

www.ingramcontent.com/pod-product-compliance
Lightning Source LLC
Chambersburg PA
CBHW060704280326
41933CB00012B/2293